My Physical Therapy

I0448148

Setting Goals

Making Plans

Achieving Milestones

Celebrating Success

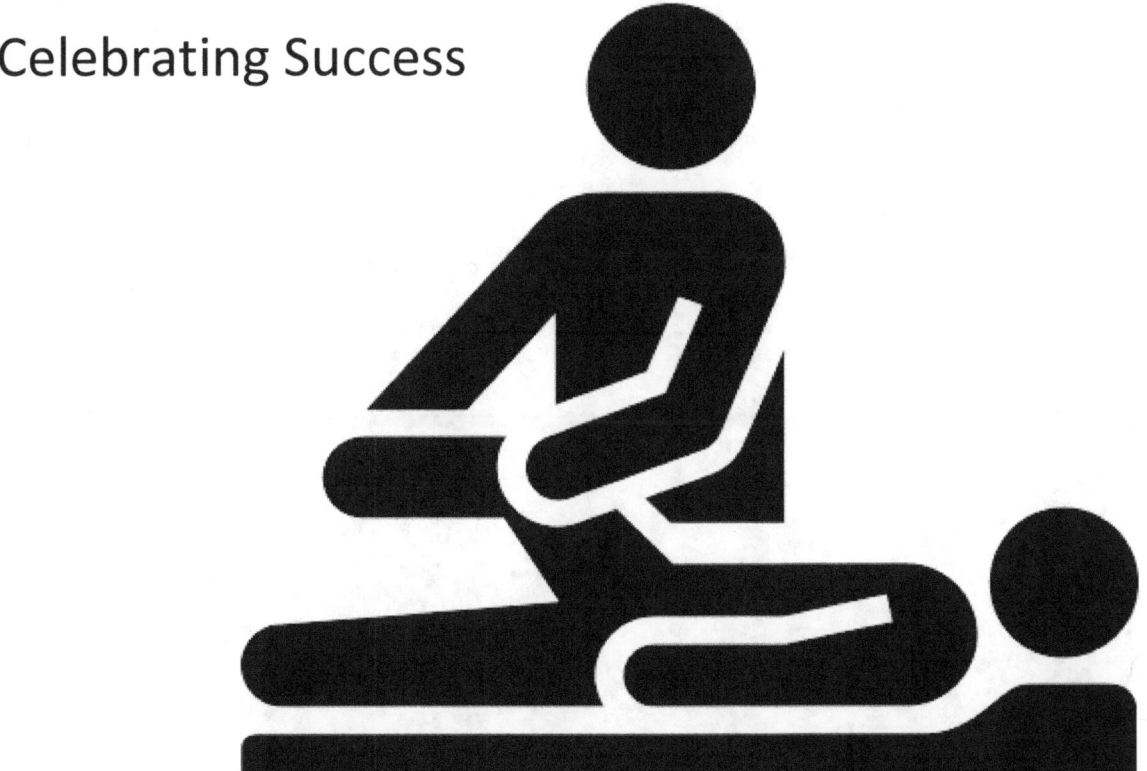

Use this journal to record your exercise routines, increase your accountability in completing assignments, and to help you celebrate the victories in your physical therapy.

My Physical Therapy

Genuine Journals
P.O. Box 813
Olympia, WA 98507
GenuineJournals.com

ISBN-13: 978-1502728654

ISBN-10: 1502728656

Table of Contents

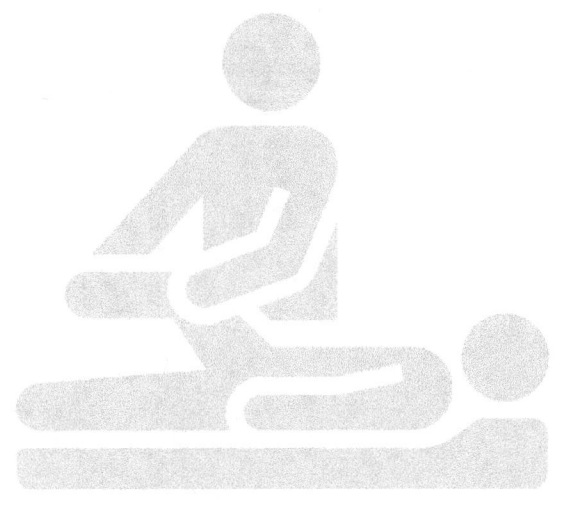

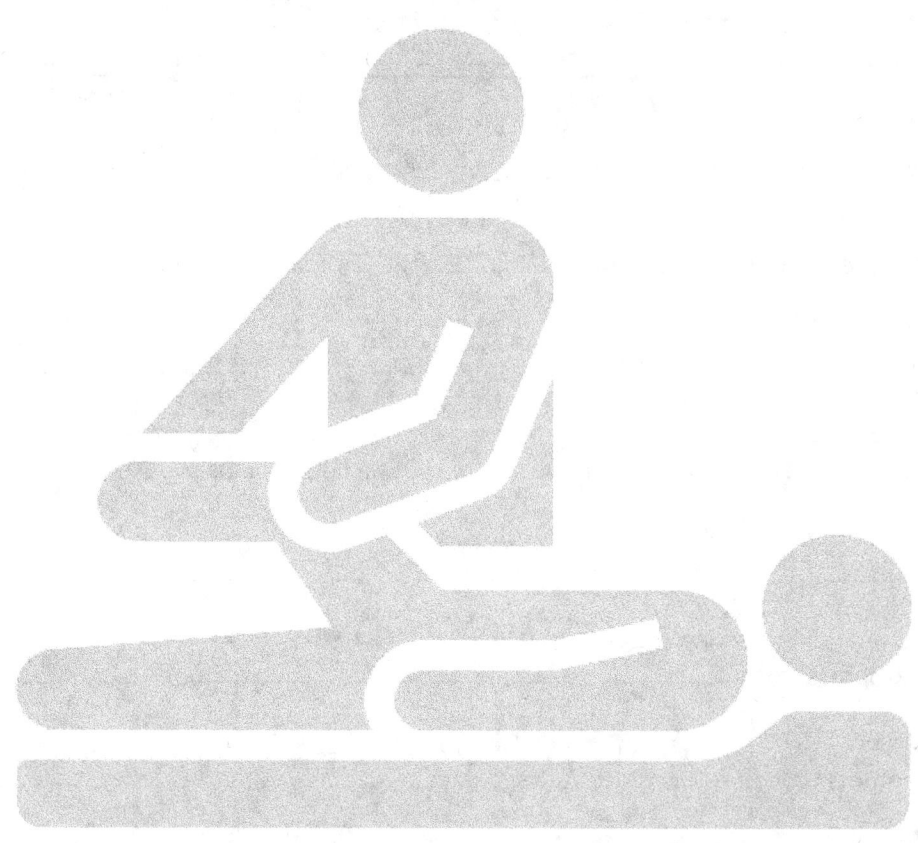

How to Use This Book

Life is a journey. And when you are recovering from a serious injury that journey can be long and difficult. The road can be made shorter when you faithfully complete your assigned physical therapy exercises, and when you focus on and celebrate your achievements. This book will help you plot your path on that journey.

Meet with your Physical Therapist to create your exercise plan. It is valuable for both of you to know what the assigned exercises are and how faithfully you are doing them. It is also helpful to make an agreement with the Physical Therapist about how often you will meet together. Faithfully keeping a journal and completing your assignments may result in fewer visits to the therapist, and that can save you some time and money. Bring this journal to your therapy sessions. Show your therapist your exercise records and discuss your notes. Take notes on new assignments as you make progress.

Describe the Problem
What happened to make you need physical therapy? Briefly describe the injuries and surgeries that brought you into physical therapy. Your Physical Therapist may refer to this as your Problem Statement.

Record Your Assessments
Your first physical therapy session will include some measurements of your strength, range of motion, and physical abilities. Ask your therapist to describe the assessment to you, or to include it in the notes he or she gives you in the end of visit summary. Make note of any measurements of strength or range of motion. If the therapist scores or ranks you on some type of scale (such as saying you score 4 out of 5 on his/her assessment scale), write it down in your assessments section.

There will be additional assessments as therapy progresses. This is done to measure progress. Take notes on each new assessment and record them in your journal. Seeing your progress is encouraging.

Set Your Goals
What are your goals for physical therapy? When will you know you are done?

- I want to walk without a cane.
- I want to walk without limping.
- I want to drive my own car.
- I want to be able to take a shower and dress myself.
- I want to run without pain.
- I need to climb a flight of stairs without assistance.
- I want to maintain range of motion in lower extremities.
- Walk the dog around the block.
- Feel well enough to do housework or gardening.
- Run a half or full marathon.
- Return to my favorite sport.

Work with your therapist to set realistic goals. Good goals will help both of you be able to determine when therapy has concluded and you are able to continue on your own.

Define Your Routine

Your therapist will assign activities or exercises for you to complete. You may be asked to do a set of several exercises every day, every other day, or a certain number of times each week. These exercise assignments will change as your strength returns and you make progress in therapy. The major portion of this book is devoted to recording what your exercises are and how often you complete them.

Many therapists will print illustrated exercise instructions and hand them to you to take home. You can stack them inside the back cover of this book so that you always have those instructions organized in a handy location. You may use those instructions to write out a few notes about how an exercise or activity is to be performed.

Write down the date every time you complete your daily assignment. There is space to make notes about your workout. You may want to note how many repetitions you were able to do, any pain you may have encountered, or if you had to stop early and why.

Celebrate Your Achievements

Focus on the things you can do today that you couldn't do yesterday. If we constantly focus on the things we can't do, we can become sad. Keeping a journal of your achievements in your recovery can be very encouraging.

In the early stages of recovery you may find new things that you can do every day that you could not do the day before. Write them down even if they seem small or trivial. You will thank yourself later when you review your journal and you want to see how far you have come.

These milestones may be farther apart as your recovery continues. After a while you will be noticing new things every week that you weren't doing the week before. It may be a new activity you can do, or it just might be a decrease in your pain medication dosage. This is your chance to celebrate the small things. They will add up!

Problem Statement

Describe the injuries and surgeries that brought you into physical therapy.

_____

_____

_____

_____

_____

_____

_____

_____

_____

_____

_____

_____

_____

_____

_____

_____

_____

_____

_____

_____

_____

_____

_____

_____

_____

_____

_____

Problem Statement

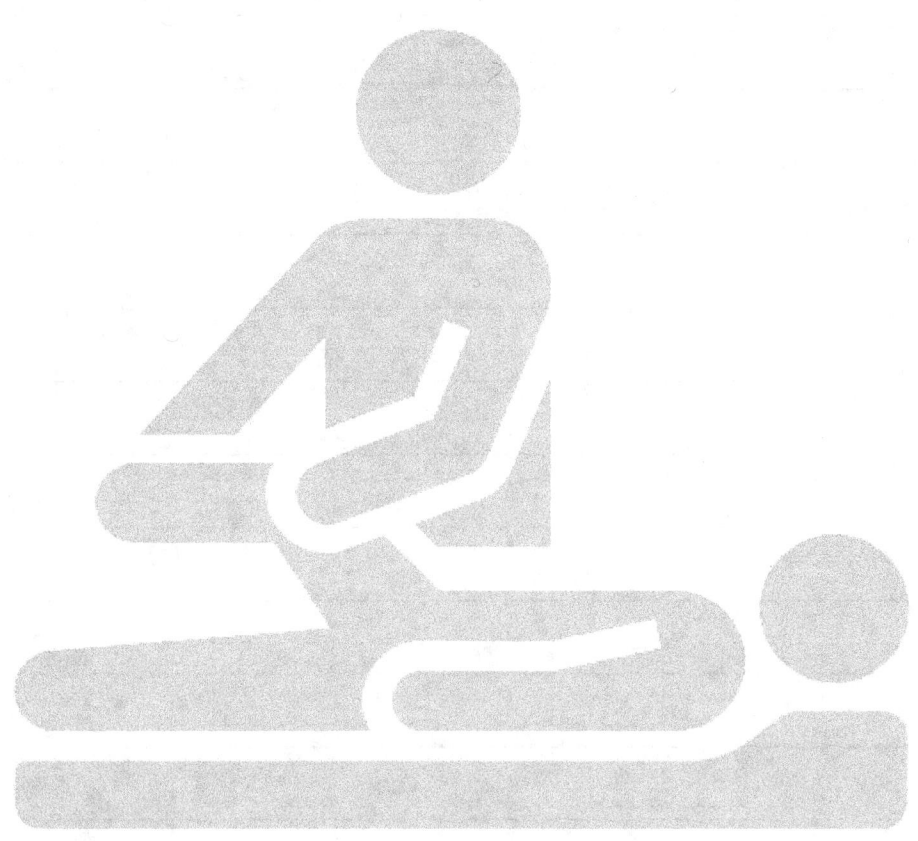

Assessments

Record a summary of the assessments made by your Physical Therapist.

Therapist	Date

Assessment

Therapist	Date

Assessment

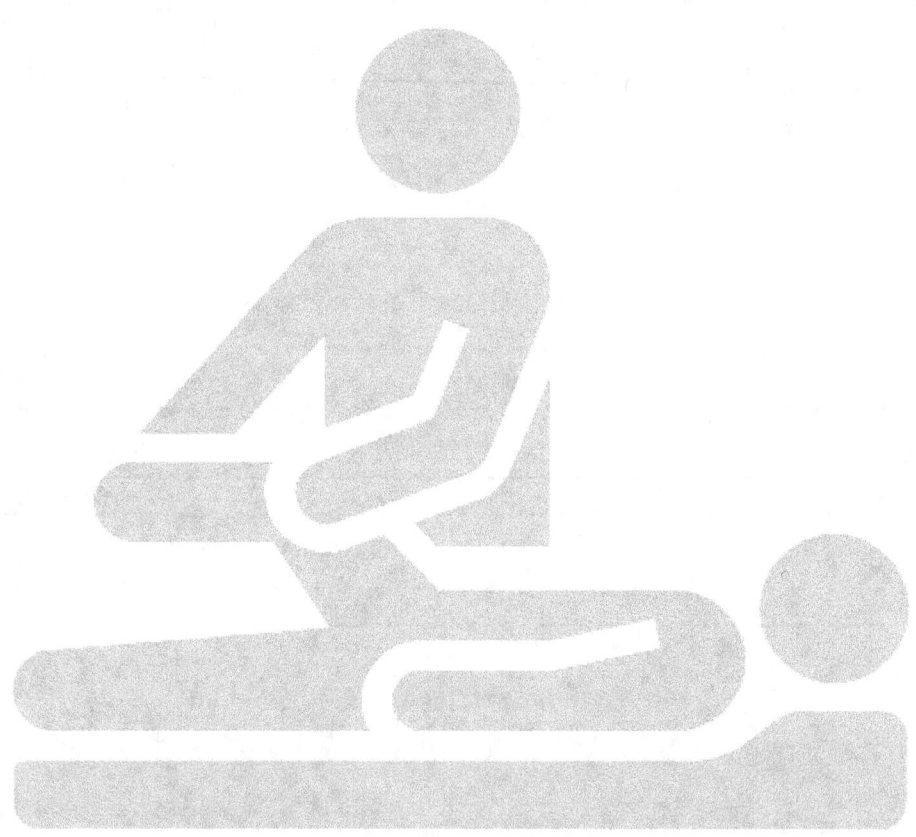

Assessments

Record a summary of the assessments made by your Physical Therapist.

Therapist	Date

Assessment

Therapist	Date

Assessment

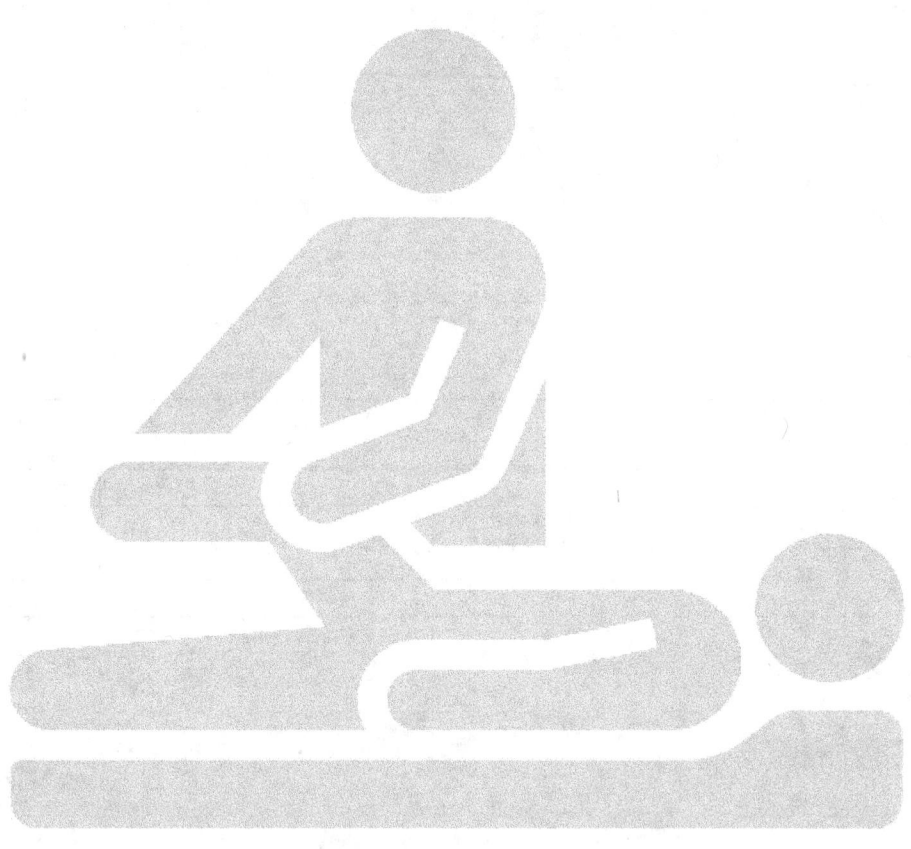

Goals

What are the things you hope to achieve through physical therapy? What types of measures or activities will help you know when you are finished with your therapy program? Goals may change over time, and new goals may emerge as therapy progresses.

Physical Therapy Goal
Target Date:

Physical Therapy Goal
Target Date:

Physical Therapy Goal
Target Date:

Physical Therapy Goal
Target Date:

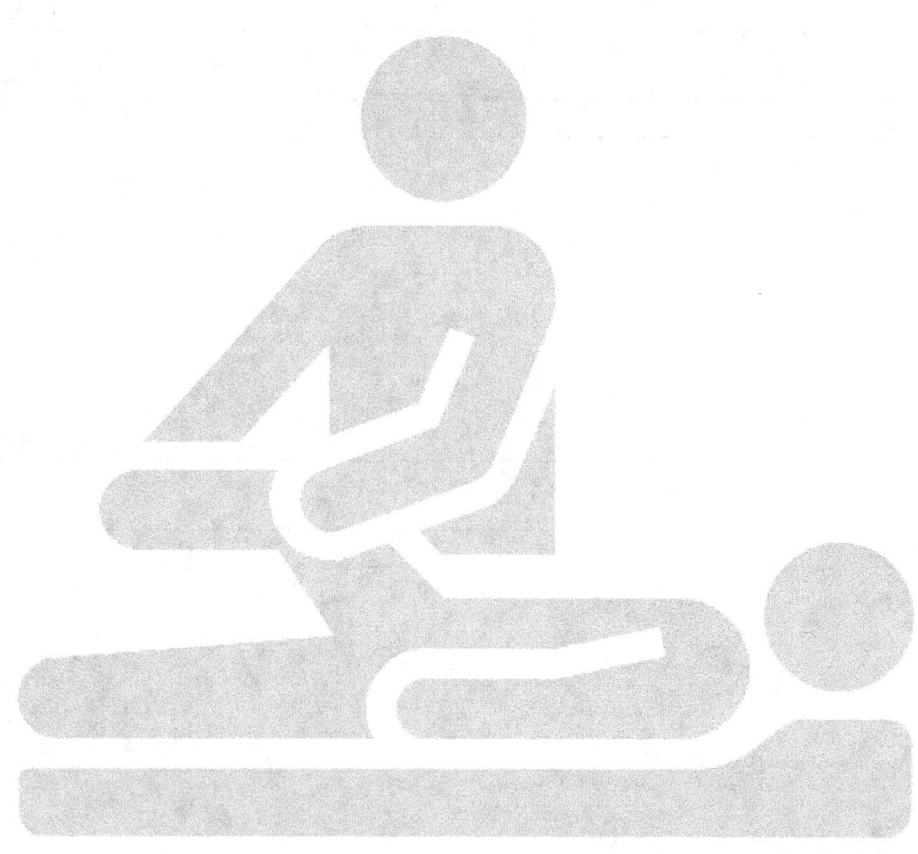

Goals

What are the things you hope to achieve through physical therapy? What types of measures or activities will help you know when you are finished with your therapy program? Goals may change over time, and new goals may emerge as therapy progresses.

Physical Therapy Goal
Target Date:

Physical Therapy Goal
Target Date:

Physical Therapy Goal
Target Date:

Physical Therapy Goal
Target Date:

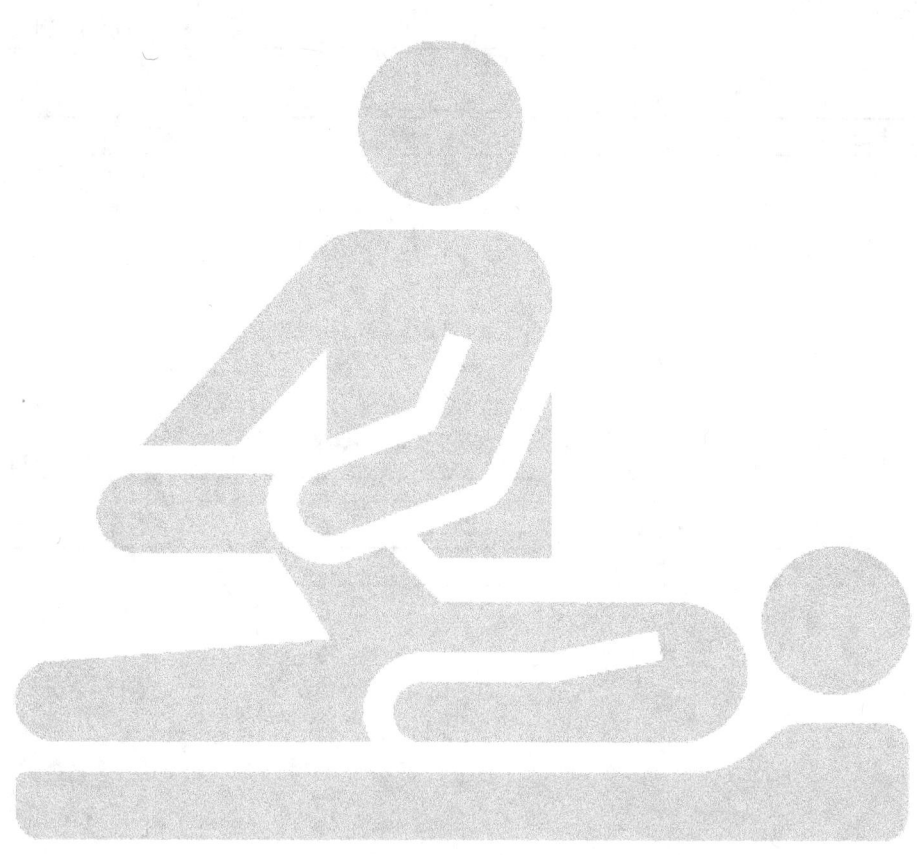

Assignments and Progress Notes

Name each assigned activity or exercise; describe how the activity is performed and how frequently it is to be done.

Exercise/Activity Name:	Date:

Instructions:

Date:	Remark:	Date:	Remark:

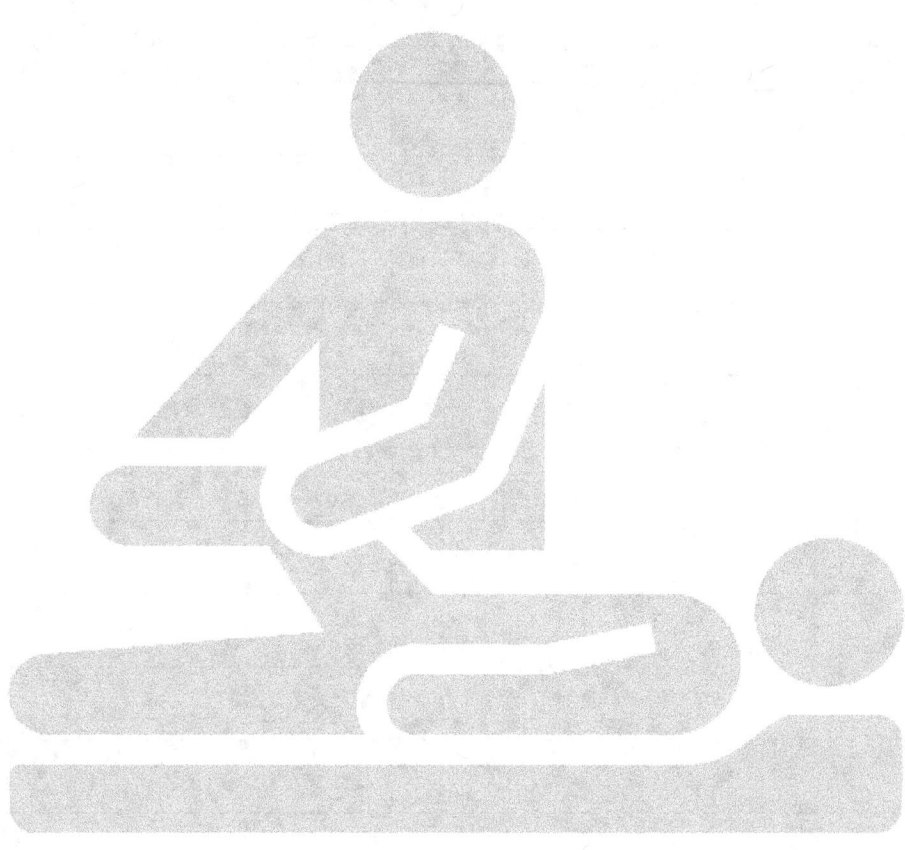

Assignments and Progress Notes

Name each assigned activity or exercise; describe how the activity is performed and how frequently it is to be done.

Exercise/Activity Name:	Date:
Instructions:	

Date:	Remark:	Date:	Remark:

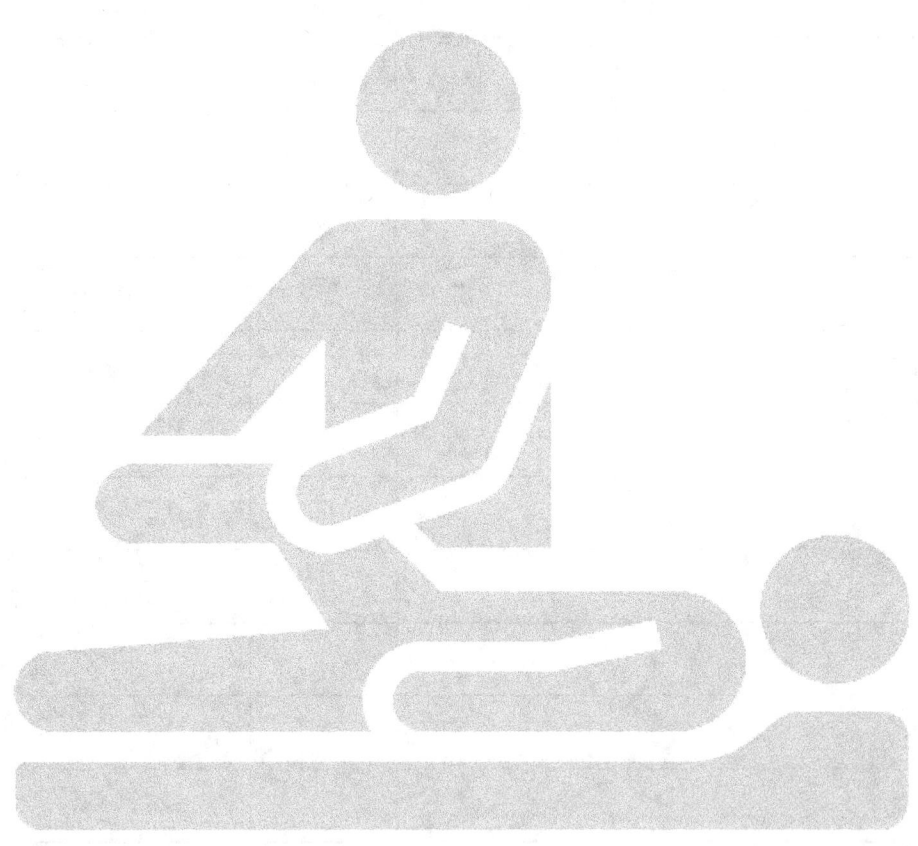

Assignments and Progress Notes

Name each assigned activity or exercise; describe how the activity is performed and how frequently it is to be done.

Exercise/Activity Name:	Date:

Instructions:

Date:	Remark:	Date:	Remark:

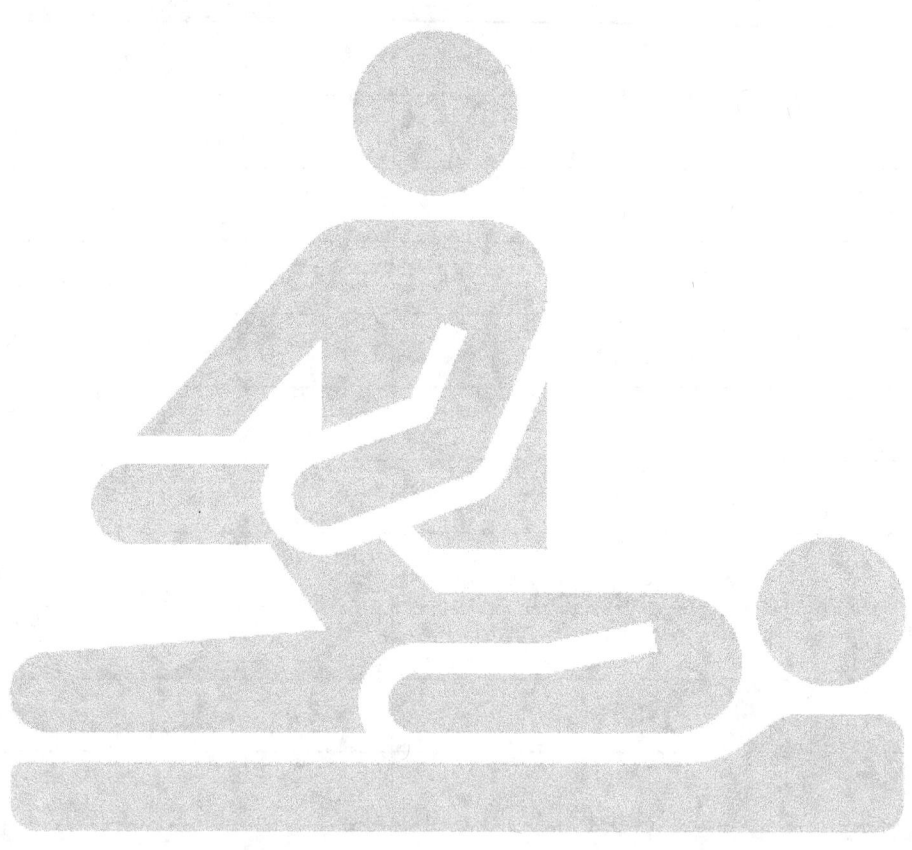

Assignments and Progress Notes

Name each assigned activity or exercise; describe how the activity is performed and how frequently it is to be done.

Exercise/Activity Name:	Date:

Instructions:

Date:	Remark:	Date:	Remark:

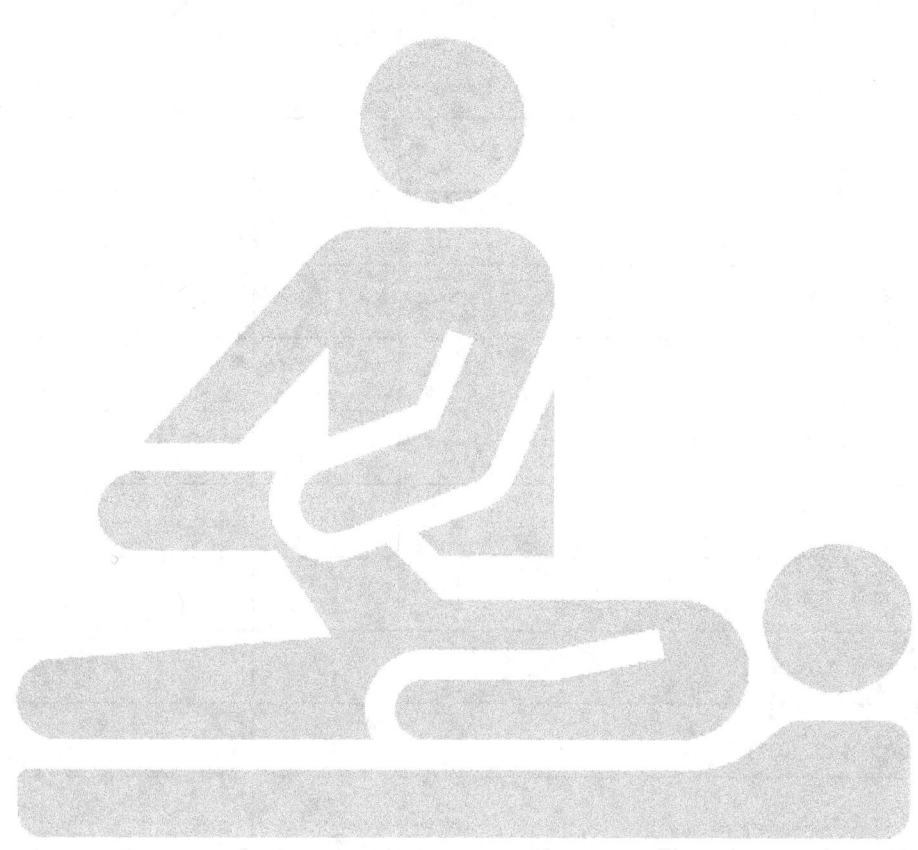

Assignments and Progress Notes

Name each assigned activity or exercise; describe how the activity is performed and how frequently it is to be done.

Exercise/Activity Name:	Date:

Instructions:

Date:	Remark:	Date:	Remark:

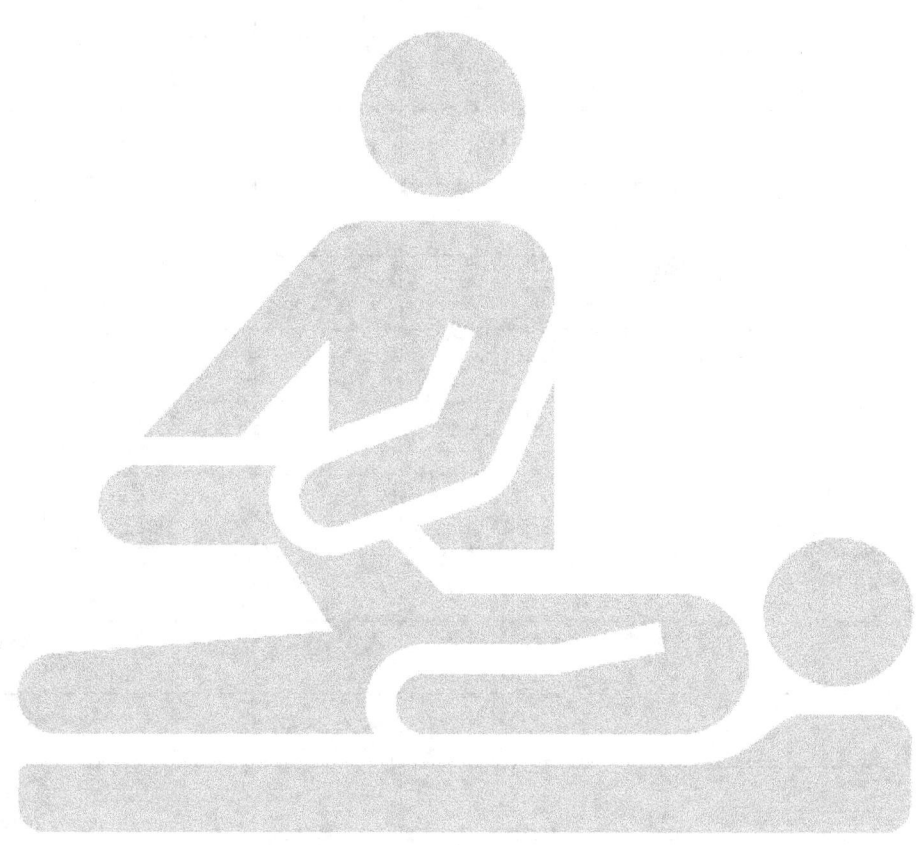

Assignments and Progress Notes

Name each assigned activity or exercise; describe how the activity is performed and how frequently it is to be done.

Exercise/Activity Name:	Date:

Instructions:

Date:	Remark:	Date:	Remark:

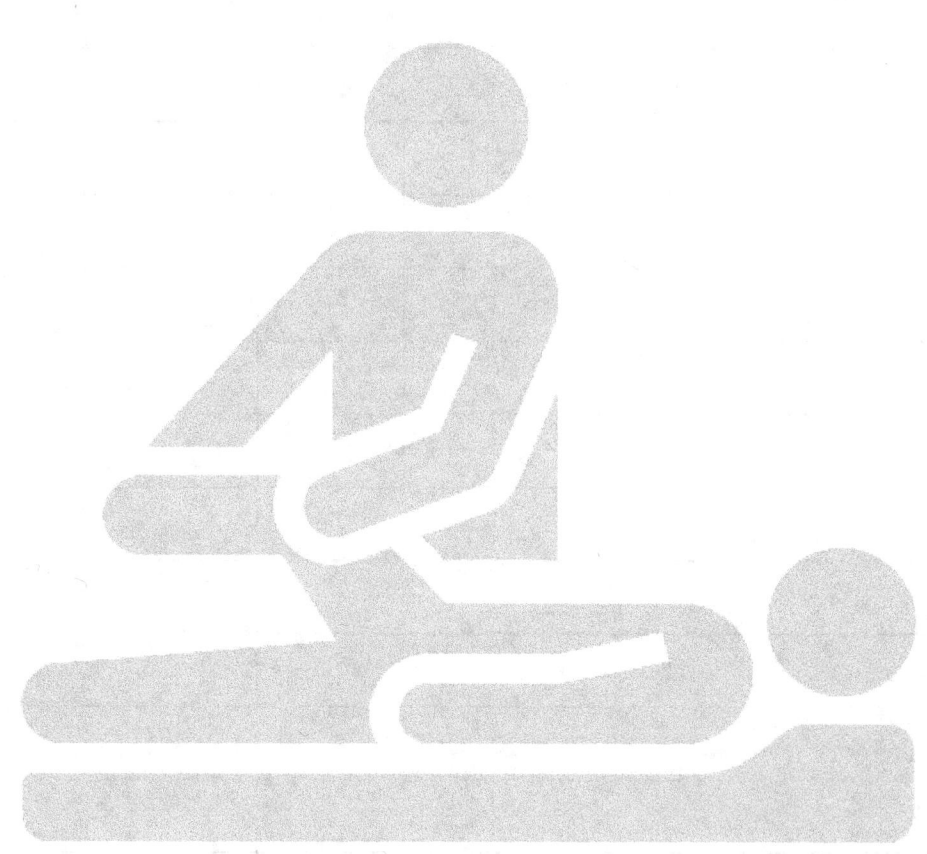

Assignments and Progress Notes

Name each assigned activity or exercise; describe how the activity is performed and how frequently it is to be done.

Exercise/Activity Name:	Date:

Instructions:

Date:	Remark:	Date:	Remark:

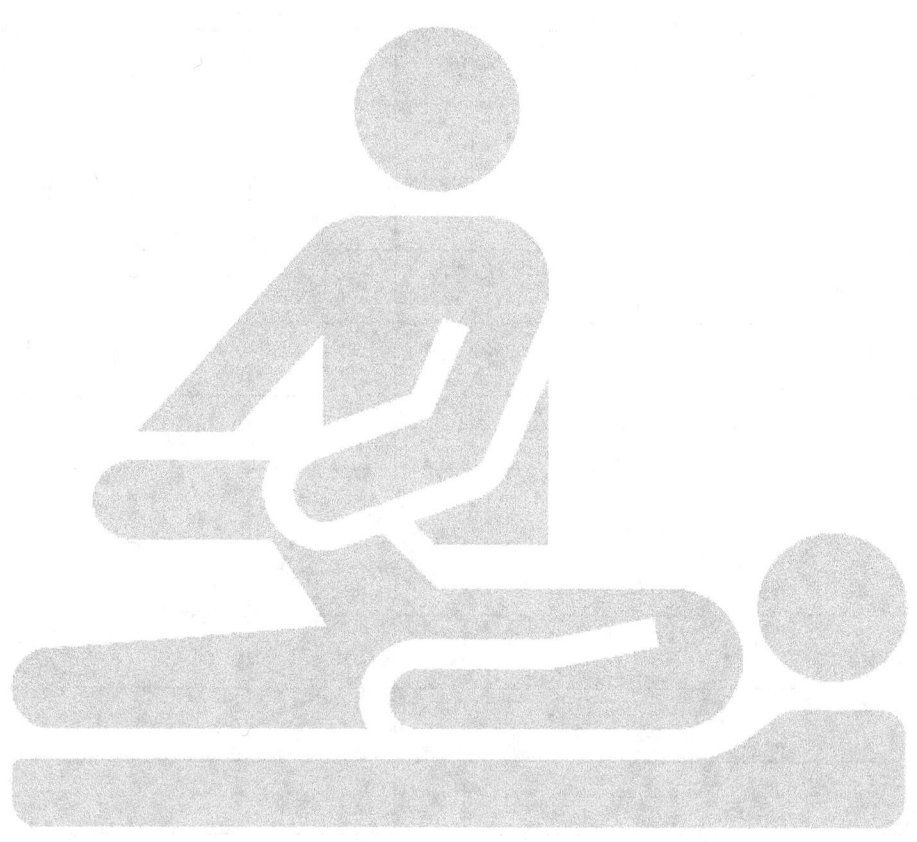

Assignments and Progress Notes

Name each assigned activity or exercise; describe how the activity is performed and how frequently it is to be done.

Exercise/Activity Name:	Date:

Instructions:

Date:	Remark:	Date:	Remark:

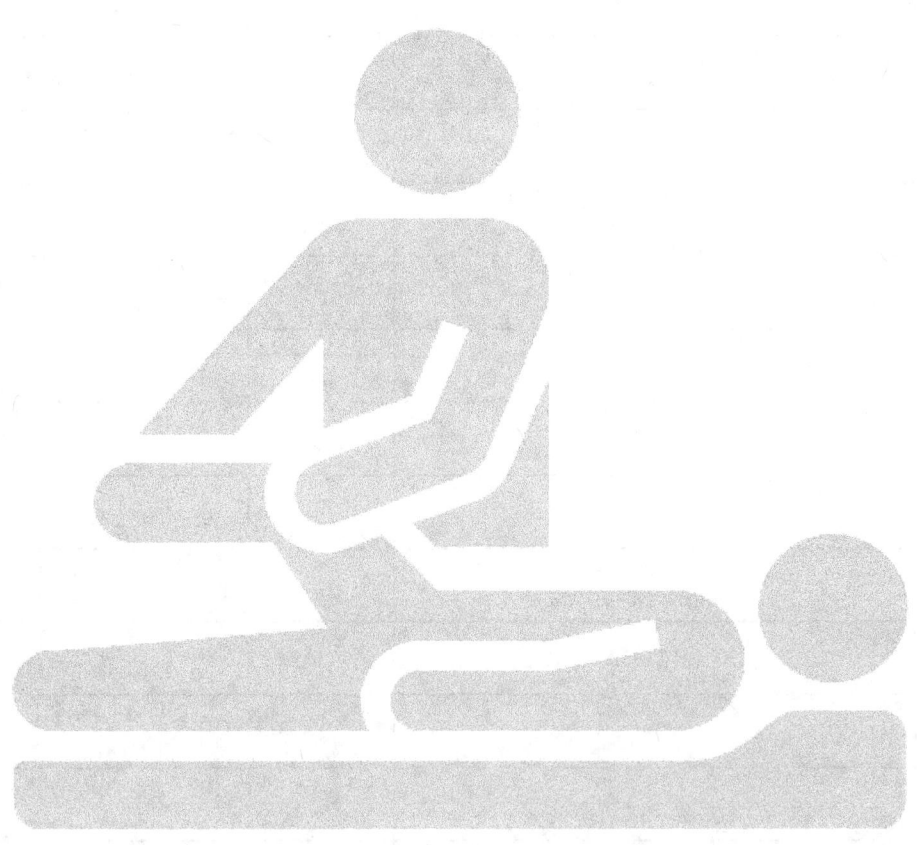

Assignments and Progress Notes

Name each assigned activity or exercise; describe how the activity is performed and how frequently it is to be done.

Exercise/Activity Name:	Date:
Instructions:	

Date:	Remark:	Date:	Remark:

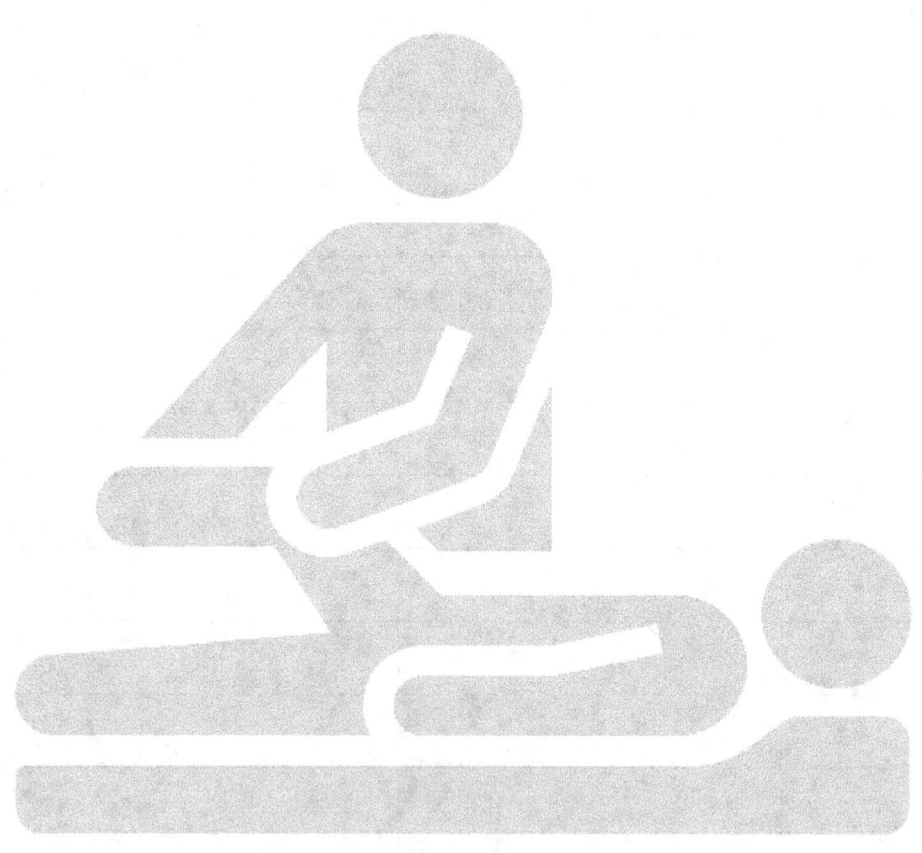

Assignments and Progress Notes

Name each assigned activity or exercise; describe how the activity is performed and how frequently it is to be done.

Exercise/Activity Name:	Date:

Instructions:

Date:	Remark:	Date:	Remark:

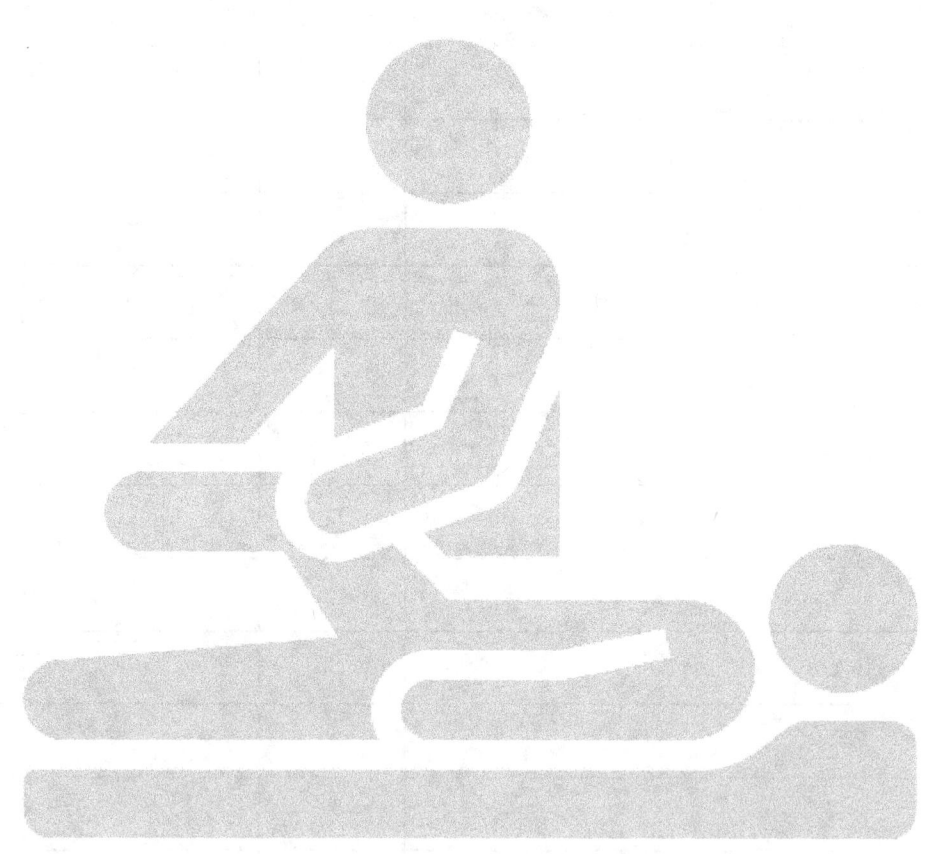

Assignments and Progress Notes

Name each assigned activity or exercise; describe how the activity is performed and how frequently it is to be done.

Exercise/Activity Name:	Date:
Instructions:	

Date:	Remark:	Date:	Remark:

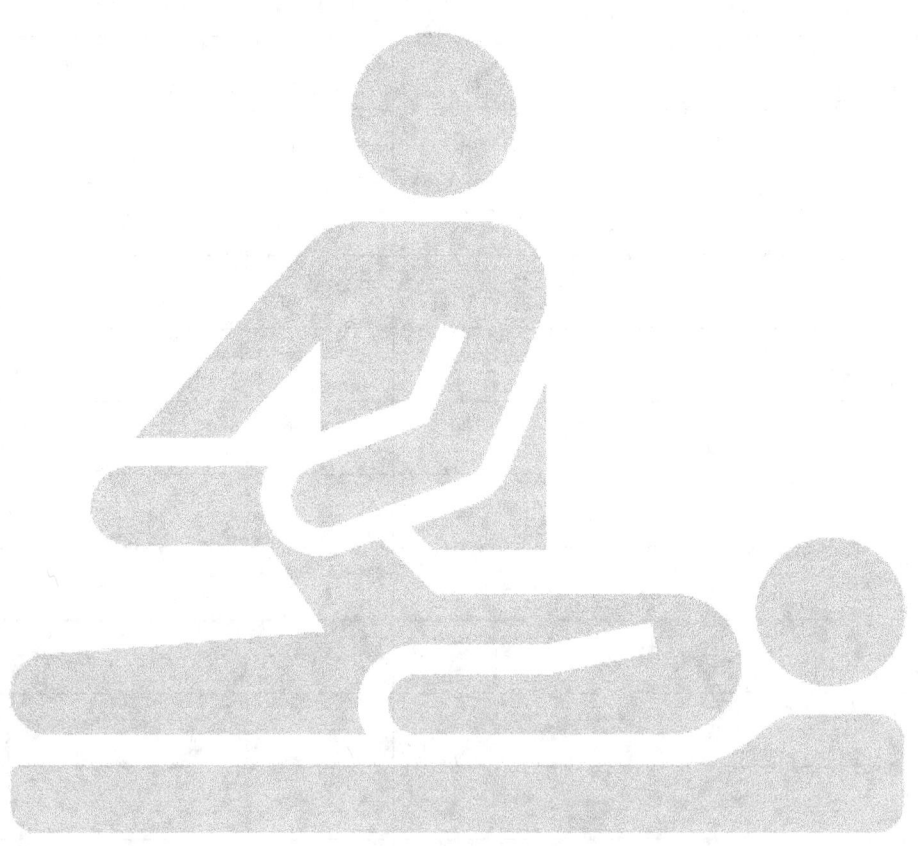

Assignments and Progress Notes

Name each assigned activity or exercise; describe how the activity is performed and how frequently it is to be done.

Exercise/Activity Name:	Date:
Instructions:	

Date:	Remark:	Date:	Remark:

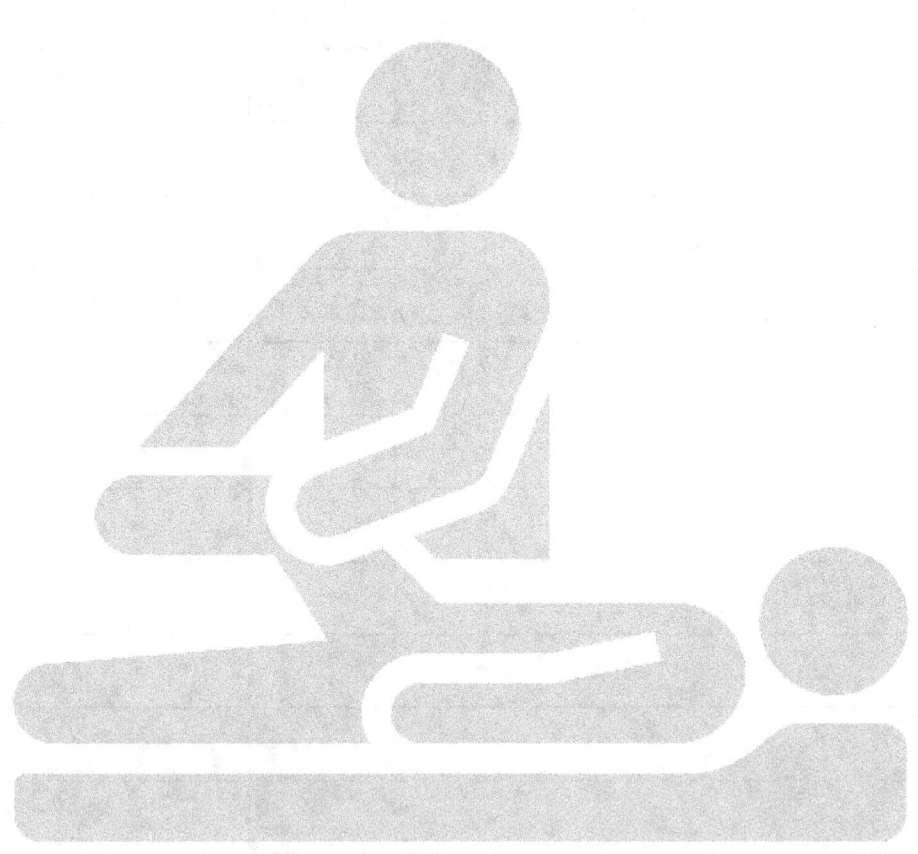

Celebrate Achievements

Make note of all those little things that show your progress.

Date:	Achievement:

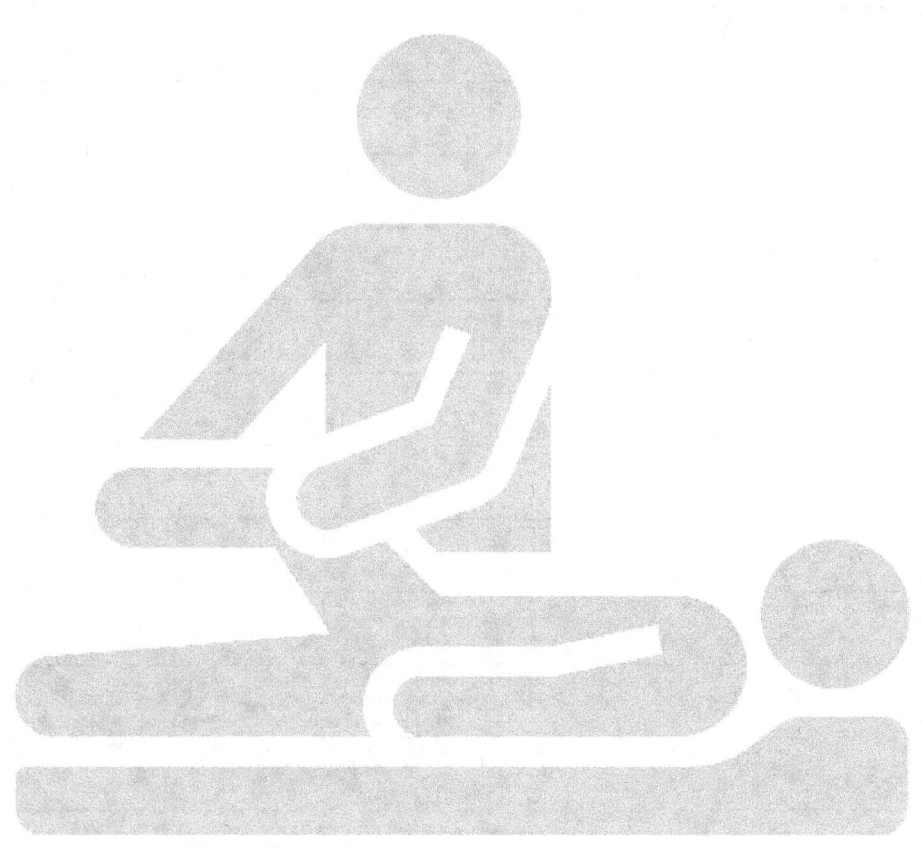

Celebrate Achievements

Make note of all those little things that show your progress.

Date:	Achievement:

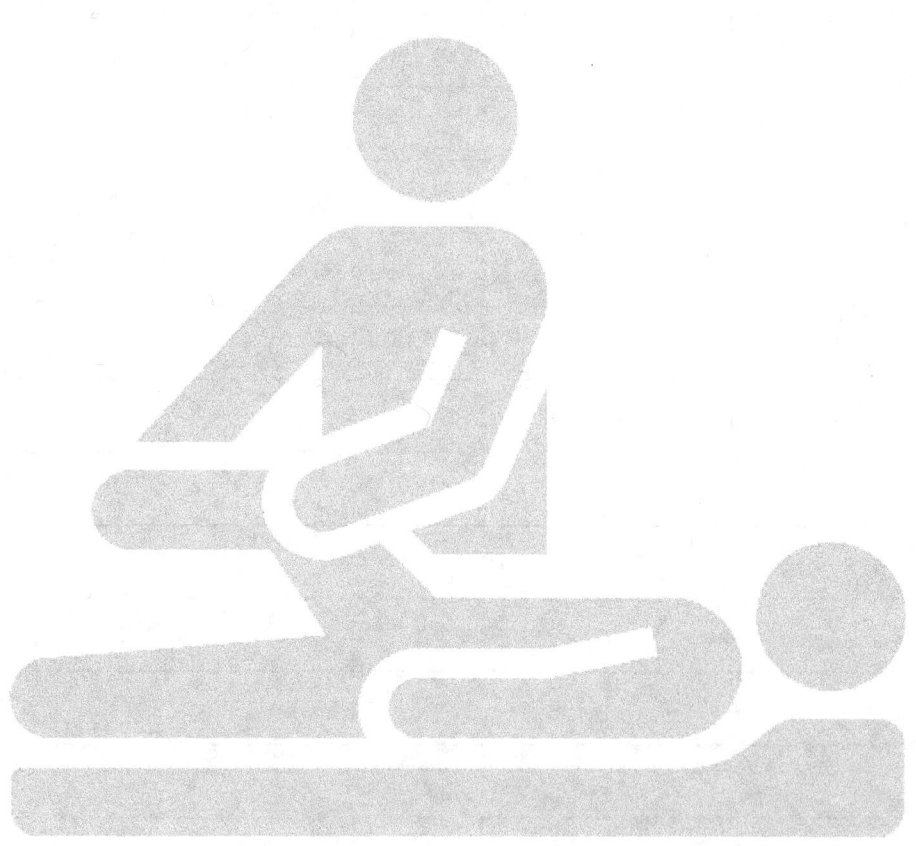

Celebrate Achievements

Make note of all those little things that show your progress.

Date:	Achievement:

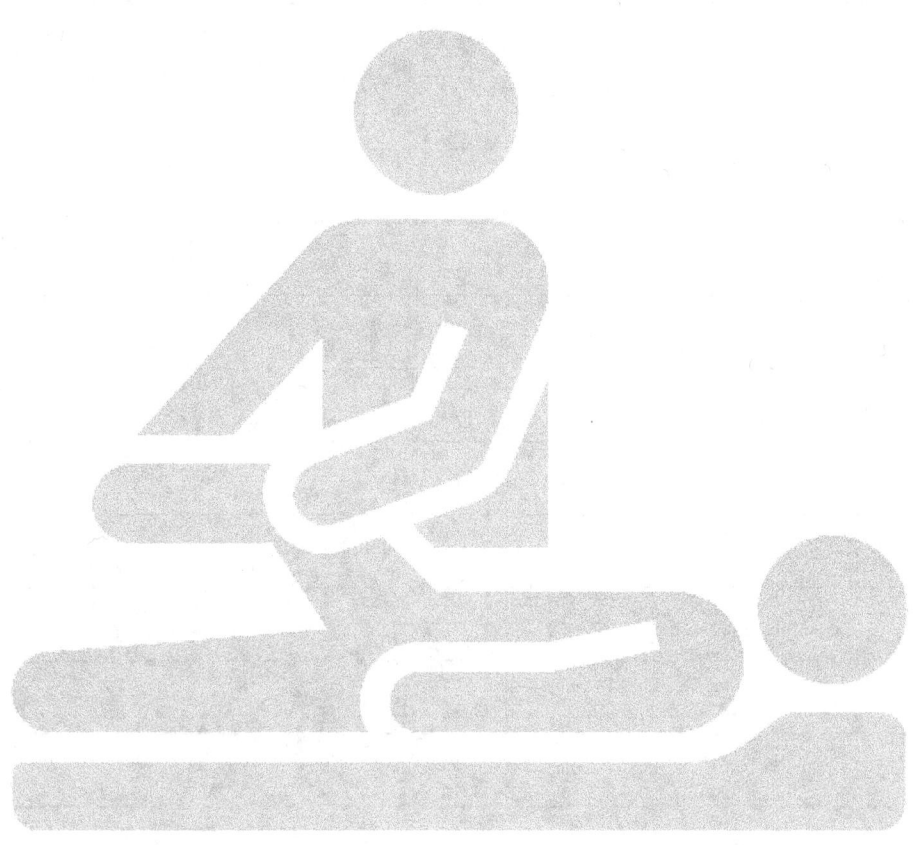

Celebrate Achievements

Make note of all those little things that show your progress.

Date:	Achievement:

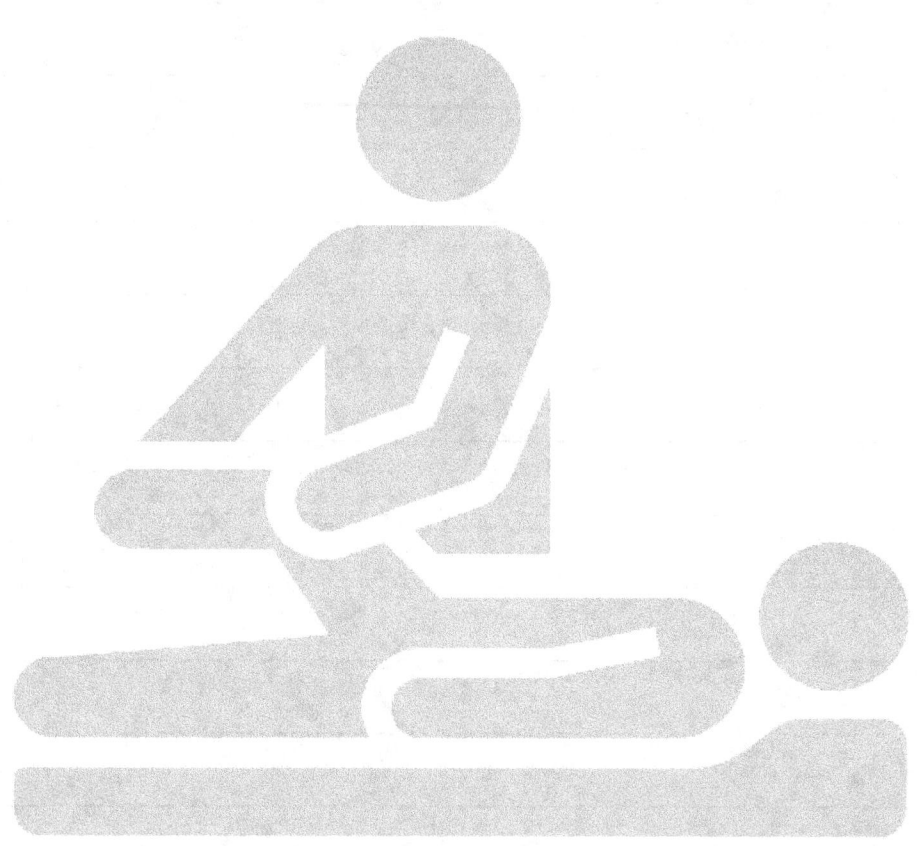